Introduction to Fats and Oils

Cooking Fats and Oils for Good Health

Health Learning Series

Dueep J. Singh

Mendon Cottage Books

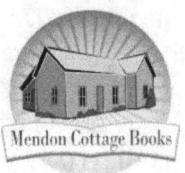

JD-Biz Publishing

Disclaimer

The information is this book is provided for informational purposes only. It is not intended to be used and medical advice or a substitute for proper medical treatment by a qualified health care provider. The information is believed to be accurate as presented based on research by the author.

The contents have not been evaluated by the U.S. Food and Drug Administration or any other Government or Health Organization and the contents in this book are not to be used to treat cure or prevent disease.

The author or publisher is not responsible for the use or safety of any diet, procedure or treatment mentioned in this book. The author or publisher is not responsible for errors or omissions that may exist.

Warning

The Book is for informational purposes only and before taking on any diet, treatment or medical procedure, it is recommended to consult with your primary health care provider.

Check out some of the other Healthy Gardening Series books at Amazon.com

Gardening Series on Amazon

Check out some of the other Health Learning Series books at Amazon.com

Health Learning Series on Amazon

Table of Contents

Introduction

Why would anybody want to write a book on fats and oils, especially when they are used in cooking, you may ask. This is because most of us have a mindset that fats and oils in our food are definitely items to be avoided by any sensible person who is bothered about the state of his health.

Well, the answer is that that we have become so obsessed about weight loss and weight gain, that we have forgotten one main medical truth. Our body cannot do without fat, and that is the reason why any diet which talks about 0% fat is not going to be helpful to our bodies.

That is because our bodies are genetically and naturally programmed to have a layer of subcutaneous fat, which we normally call cellulite. That is to protect the inner organs from any sort of damage from external sources, and it is between the skin, the muscle and the inner organs.

The vulnerable inner organs, especially in the stomach region are protected with this layer – the obese layer you call a beer belly – and that is why any fatty item you eat is going to be observed by your body and the fatty cells turned into "protective" cellulite.

For millenniums, this fatty layer was considered to be a storehouse of energy, from which the body could get extra nutrition. When human beings were in a state of starvation or malnutrition due to the paucity of food, the fatty cells would break up and provide them with the necessary energy in order to keep going until the natural fat storage layer could be restored again with available food.

But as time went by, people had easy access to food, and that is what made them believe that that extra fatty layer was unsightly, ungainly, and not so beautiful. Remember that this is a relatively modern concept, started in the West, because even now, the concept of beautiful in many parts of the world, including Asia, Africa and the Middle East is a body with the 3 B's – bosom, belly and behind, for women.

In the same manner, even up to the medieval times, the idea of a beautiful lady was a Ruben – esque plump beauty, who had spent most of her life, dining off cream, butter and carbohydrate-based items.

Men who were fat were considered to be prosperous because they were able to afford to eat enough of fatty food. They were not lean, mean, fighting machines because they just lay back on their couches and order their warriors to go hunt up meals for them. That is why many of the portraits you see of the aristocrats of old are going to be of fat men surrounded by protective lean bodyguards.

Even now, in many parts of the world, the idea of being fat is synonymous with prosperity, good eating and even beauty.

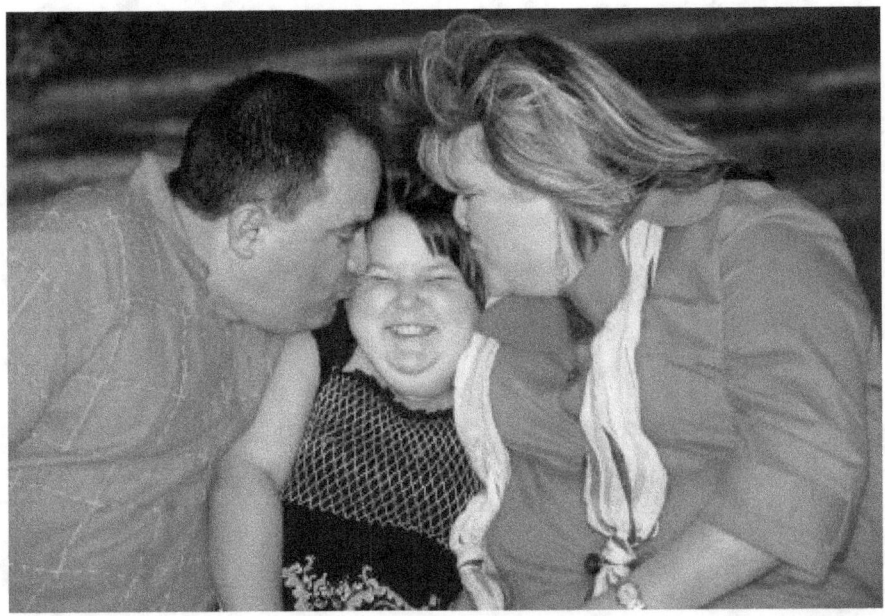

However, in the West, with its two World Wars, which brought the population of a majority of the countries to near starvation level, the idea of being completely thin became an obsession. And that is why more and more folks stopped using healthy fat to cook food and instead started using chemical-based products or artificial products like margarine insert of natural foodstuffs.

Besides this, a caloric imbalance is the reason why people suffer from obesity and overweight. This means that you are expending too few calories in the form of "burning off calories" in proportion to the amounts of calories eaten in your diet. Also, environmental, behavioral, genetic and dietary factors are going to influence your health, possibly causing obesity and overweight problems.

This book is for all those people who want to know more about oils and fats and their nutritive value. If you are obsessed with absolutely no fat in your diet, because your colleagues, mama, best friend, or somebody endorsing a weight loss diet, told you that, just think a little.

Why has fat been an important part of the 4 food groups? That is because it is necessary to keep your body healthy and functioning properly.

So let us start with-

Butter

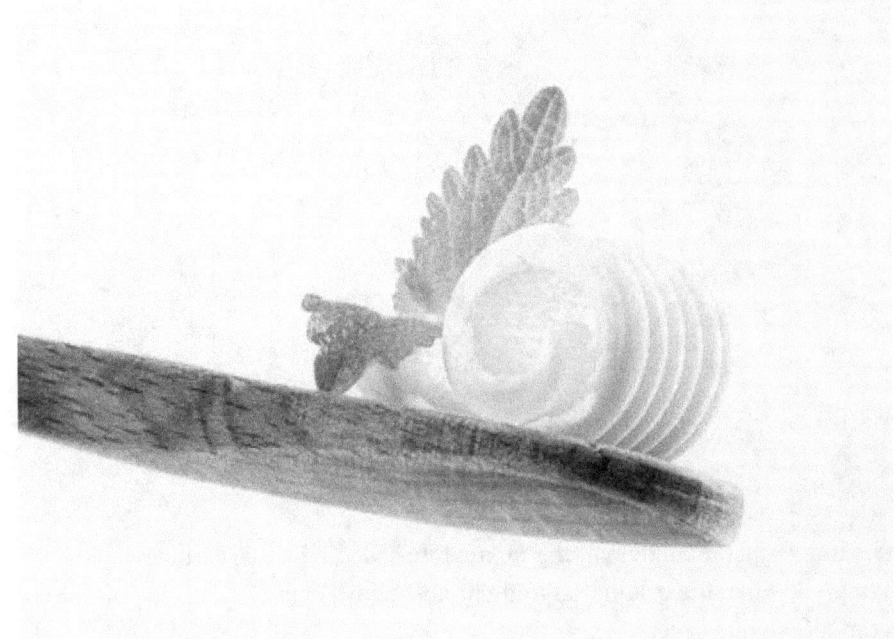

Butter is probably the most digestible and nutritious of all the fats, and has been in existence for millenniums. Not only has it been an important part of cookery, but it has also been used as a natural healing ingredient, down the ages.

This is the most popular of fats, because of its delicious taste. Julia Childs could not do without it, and plenty of it. And naturally, any Spanish, Italian and French cook would make sure that she had plenty of homemade butter ready at hand, when she was cooking up something delicious for her hungry brood.

 Its very feeble substitute, margarine may taste like butter, but it is definitely not the real stuff. Besides, margarine is an artificial manufactured product, made up of plant oils and other hydrogenated products and one cannot substitute plant oils for real butter, made out of real cow's milk.

Butter has been used as a cooking fat in all the cases where taste is of paramount experience and no other substitute is going to do.

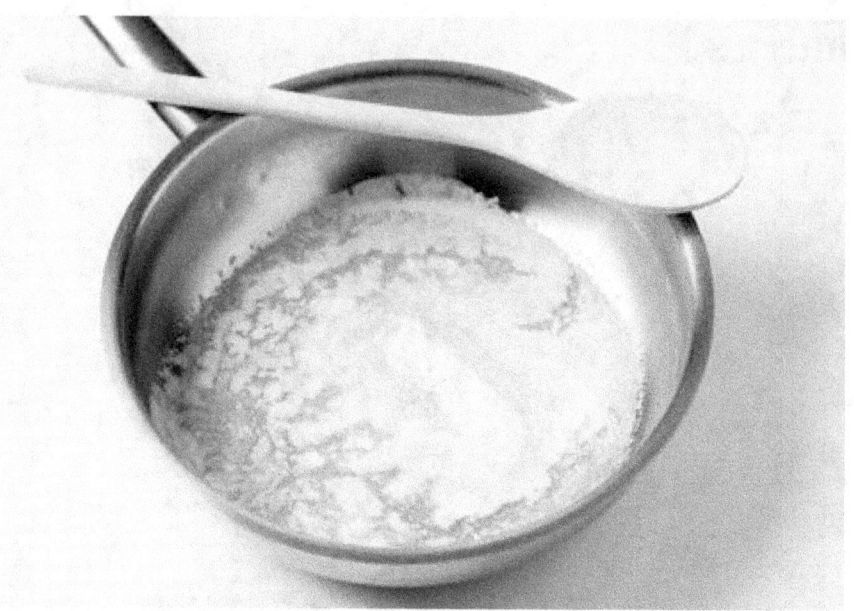

For example, just imagine making up a white sauce with margarine or with cooking oil, when the original ingredient needed was butter. This is going to be a travesty of a white sauce.

Just stir in a knob of butter into gravy or sauce after it has been cooked and you are going to get a thicker rich product with a much improved flavor and look. Many people say that dishes made up of butter are greasy and oily. That is because they have been brought up to eat totally fat-free dishes, and they have a concept of every dish with fat in it is going to be greasy.

That is not so. Have you seen layers of butter floating on the surface of the dishes you eat made up of pure butter? Butter gets assimilated in the food. It is only clarified butter, which floats on the surface.

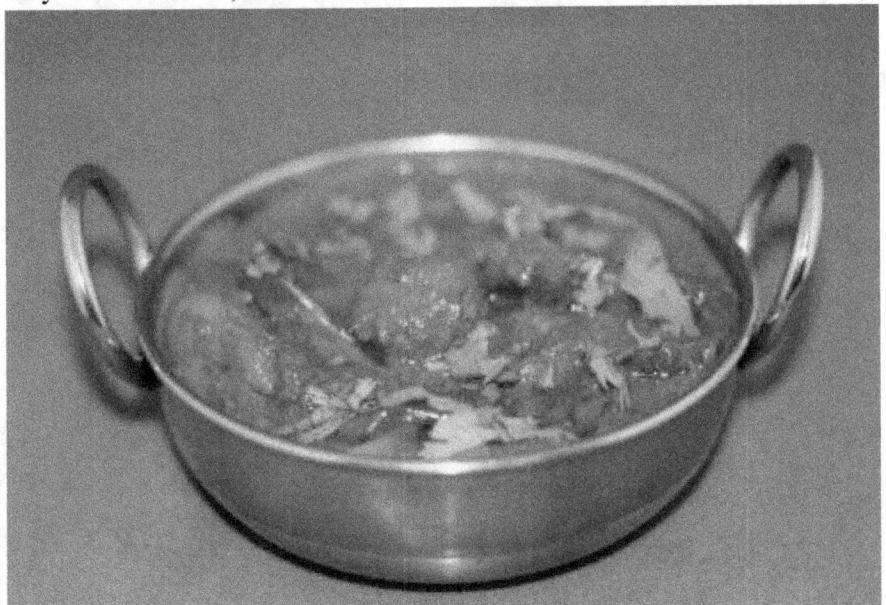

Butter chicken, one of the most globally well-known dishes of Indian cuisine is made up of chicken fried in pure butter, a rich tomato, ginger and onion sauce, spices and herbs. It is eaten only on festive and special occasions, because even though it is rich, delicious, tasty and addictive, one has gotten into the habit of not eating too much butter rich food, especially if one leads a sedentary lifestyle.

This visible layer of butter is going to be stirred into the gravy before serving and garnishing, so that you do not think you are eating rich, oily and greasy butter chicken.

Butter browns and burns so quickly that it is quite unsuitable as a frying fat, though, a little can be added to oil used for frying for the sake of the taste. Moreover, it contains 12 – 15% of water and as we know oils splutters when it is hot and if water is added to it. So you will have spluttering butter the moment it starts heating up a bit.

Nevertheless, the butter's tendency to burn becomes useful when you want a crust of pastry, crumbs and potatoes which have to be browned in the oven or under the grill. This is going to give you a buttery glaze. Brushing the surface with a little bit of butter, before grilling is going to achieve this purpose.

What Is Clarified Butter?

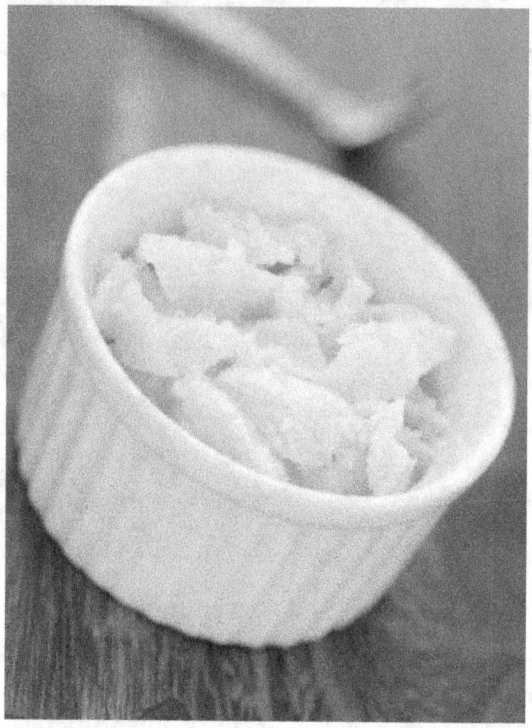

Now this is butter in its purest and most concentrated form. Dietitians will call this pure poison, because of its fat content. But gourmets beg to differ, because they consider any food made in clarified butter to be fit for the Gods.

Caloric imbalance is the reason why people suffer from obesity and overweight. This means that you are expending too few calories in the form of "burning off calories" in proportion to the amounts of calories eaten in your diet. Also, environmental, behavioral, genetic and dietary factors are going to influence your health, possibly causing obesity and overweight problems.

That reminds me of an amusing statement made by one of my friends who enjoys eating and drinking well. She was going to Europe, and was looking forward to the holiday, when she would have the opportunity to eat nouvelle cuisine to her heart's delight. And then she invoked an old Eastern saying "On every grain of food has been written the Name of its Eater."

When I looked perplexed, she said that she was going to the lands of prosperity and plenty. But the people there were starving themselves on purpose because It Was Not Written In Their Fate to enjoy the bounty given to them by nature. She found it very ironical, because this was due to their own self-imposed restrictions, pertaining to calorie counting and weight loss. So they were missing out half of the fun of life, because they did not eat butter, olive oil, fats, and other delicious food items, because they were either on a dietary restriction, or they were trying to lose weight, or they had a built-in autosuggestion, telling them that that food was not healthy for them, because they had been taught that since childhood.

Well, I feel I am lucky that I was born in the East, where we eat and drink aplenty, and give thanks for what we have been given, and which we enjoy when we want.

So that is the reason why I am going to tell you about taste in the form of concentrated butter, which we call clarified butter.

This is so powerful that it is only taken in small quantities – not more than one or 2 tablespoons for a day, and only when you are not living a sedentary lifestyle. This tip is for all those calorie watchers, who were depriving themselves of delicious and tasty food, just because...

How to make Clarified Butter

Start collecting cream from your daily milk supply. 6 to 8 days, will give you enough of cream to make clarified butter, also known as Desi[1] ghee. Heat the milk cream, and you are going to find it melting into ghee. The leftover sediment is delicious, when spread on Indian breads, Pita breads, or over any spicy dish.

Villagers traditionally make Desi ghee in Asia by adding yogurt to the cream for a week or so. They intend to turn it into buttermilk, fresh butter and Desi ghee by churning. This turning process has three stages. Add water to the yoghurt cream cream mixture and you get buttermilk and butter. Heat the butter and you are going to get Desi ghee.

Desi ghee is also a very powerful healing agent. It is normally used in the making up of herbal medicines, because it is made of pure creamy milk butter. It is also used in making beauty creams, potions, lotions and other skin ointments.

It has a powerful aroma, and that is why only just a spoonful is added to fry meats. It is going to float on the surface of the meat dish, after it has been cooked, so you need to stir the gravy before serving. Also, the food is not going to taste greasy, even though it looks like it has been swimming in fat.

Desi ghee is the concentrated form of pure butter, which is heated to reduce the butter of all the impurities as well as moisture. This concentrated butter is normally used in Eastern cuisine, for searing meat, sautéing and frying food, because they offer its higher burning point.

You make this at home by taking 2 pounds of best unsalted butter and melting it in a heavy bottomed pan. Allow the butter to liquefy on low heat for about 40 minutes. Maintain this simmering point, until all of the moisture in the butter has evaporated. The impurities are going to sink to the bottom of the pan. Remember to keep stirring the butter, so that it does not burn.

---

[1] The word Desi (as in "All right, start 'splaining." Incidentally, he never said "Lucy, you got some 'splaining to do", ever!) stands for "of the country, native" here.

Pour off the clear butter and strain it through several thicknesses of muslin cloth. Clarified butter is going to last for about a year, if it is placed in a cool and dry place. This butter is exorbitantly expensive. So in the East, people with easy access to plenty of fresh milk make it right in their kitchens for crisp delicious frying results, and adding that taste of pure butter to all their dishes.

Remember to remove the sediment from the top, when you store this Desi ghee in airtight glass bottles. The sediment is delicious on breads with honey.

One tablespoonful of this highly concentrated powerful oil spread on every meal surface, including vegetables, pulses and beans – every available visible surface – and eaten every day is considered to be the reason why so many people stay healthy in the villages of Asia. This is, of course, supported with plenty of hard physical work throughout the day.

Whole-wheat flour bread or "rotis" are the staple diet of people in the Northern parts of the Indian subcontinent. You spread desi ghee on them to make them tastier. Oldsters are given these hot chapaties with one spoonful of desi ghee and honey and crumpled (*churi*) to make them easily chewable, digestible and to promote good health and longevity.

This is the reason why every single oldster in the care of his family is going to be fed, one tablespoonful of desi ghee floating over any surface of meat, or dal in his luncheon menu. This is also the secret of the longevity of so many generations of ancients – clarified butter, cream, and other pure milk products.

This clarified butter is not restricted only to South Asia. It is also an important part of Middle Eastern cuisine. It is also used to heal wounds, especially to get rid of scars, by just applying a little bit of clarified butter on the wound, and then allowing it to heal naturally.

Margarine

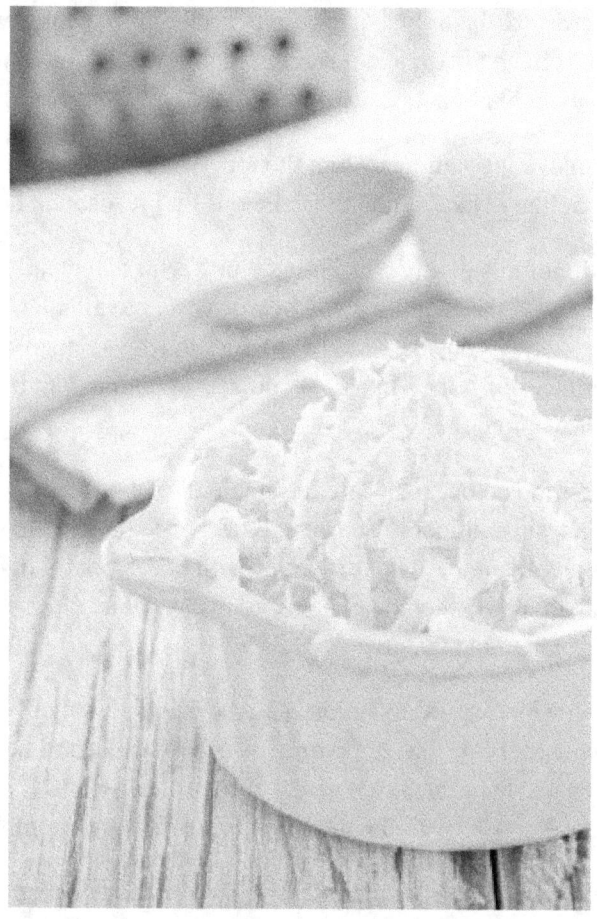

Margarine may look like butter, and is considered to be the equal of butter in every way, except of course in the matter of flavor.

Even so, the taste of margarine is remarkably pleasant. So you can use it with confidence in cake making, pastry making and for making other sweet dishes.

Margarine is now manufactured in a softened form, so it does not solidify, when you put it in the fridge like does butter. That means all you have to do is take it out from the fridge, and spread it all over your toasted bread for breakfast, instead of waiting for about 10 minutes for the butter to defrost.[2]

Margarine is also much easier to beat, with sugar than butter is. However, you can easily recognize the fact that this is not butter the moment it is melted. It is not ideal for white sauce, mashed potatoes, or hot toast.

That is why I smirk when I see a margarine advertisement, ordering me to eat margarine on freshly made toast for breakfast. I would rather see Golden butter melting on its surface.

Margarine also happens to be more economical than butter. And that is why in many countries, butter is being sold with huge amounts of margarine added to it, and sold as real butter. Also, this is not a good frying fat, because it is too watery to be used for frying.

---

[2] Incidentally, if you need to defrost frozen butter really fast, just cut it up in segments and place the glass bowl in a pan of hot water for about 3 to 4 minutes or until you see the butter melting into the consistency you prefer. This is going to speed up the defrosting process.

Lard

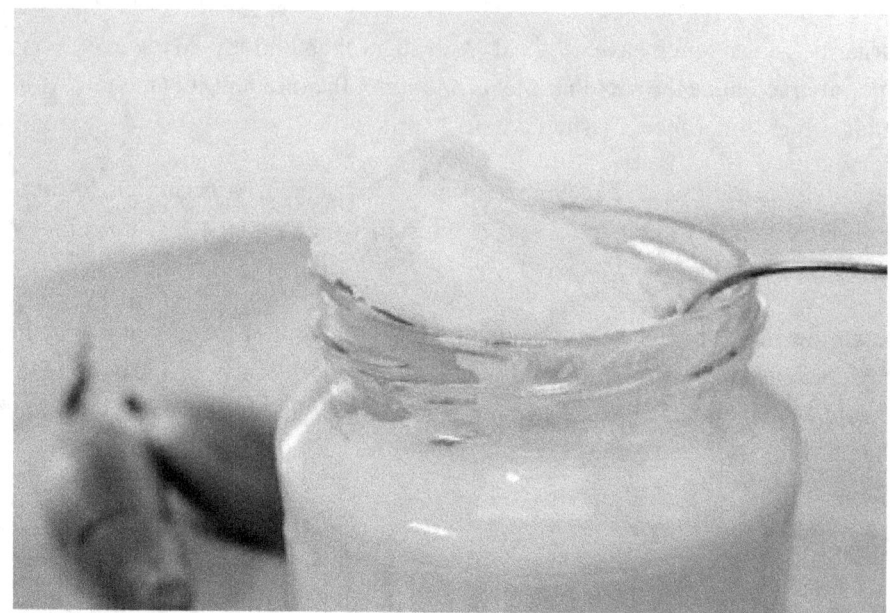

If you are lucky like me, you can get your butcher to give you fat to make pork lard. Otherwise, you will need to chop up pieces of pork fat, melt them, and strain them to make homemade lard. This process is called rendering.

Here is a very good URL, where you can see the whole process of rendering.

http://thehealthyfoodie.com/how-to-render-your-own-lard/

In days of yore, the test of a really good and efficient housewife was seen by her ability to use pork fat in order to cook food. This is the best fact, used for frying, because being hundred percent fat, it is very suitable and not at all liable to burn.

Lard has a slightly porky flavor, which is not at all unpleasant. In fact, bacon, fried in lard is tastier, I think. I know all about a very well-known pastry cook, who makes delicious fruitcake and pastry. I know his secret. He uses lard instead of any other shortening.

China, Russia, Brazil and the USA are the world's largest producers of lard, but of course the best quality lard in the world was produced in Denmark, until 1955, when local consumption began leaning towards margarine and shying away from butter.

But then we know that those Vikings of the Scandinavian countries, know all about fine eating, especially with plenty of delicious food, – think smorgasbord – accompanied with lots of high quality butter and lard. It is a pity that many of these delicious food items are now made with margarine or shortening.

Cooking Fats

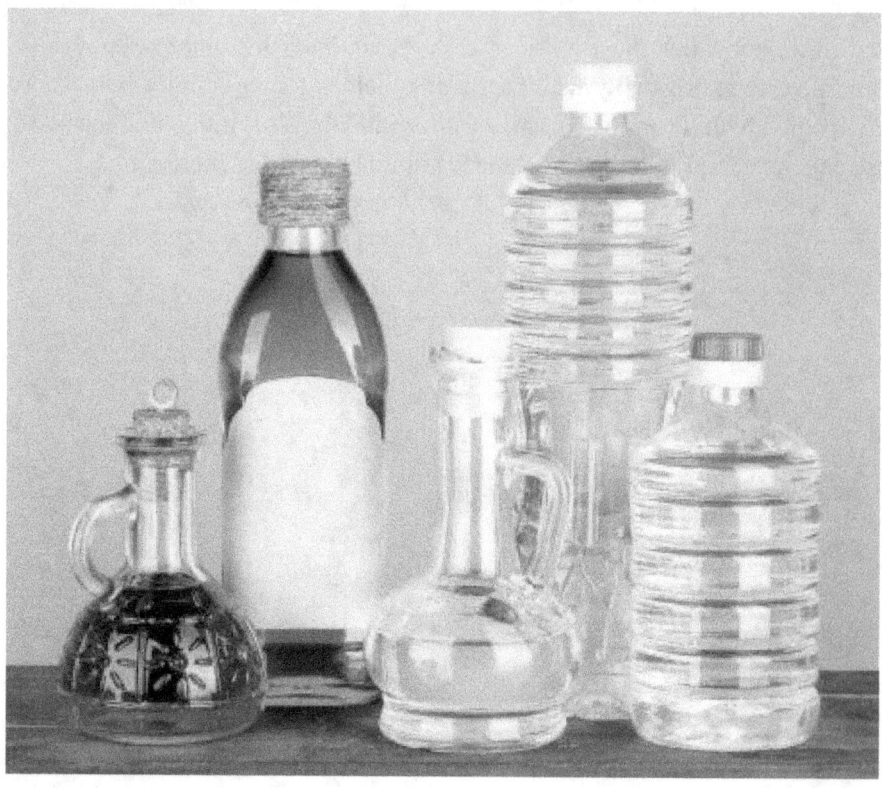

These cooking fats are the modern-day version and substitutes of supposedly healthy fats, made up of plant seed oil extracts. Many of them are marketed with the misleading label of hundred percent cholesterol free. That is because cholesterol is always caused by animal fats, including lard.

So if you are using a cooking fats, made up of corn oil or cottonseed oil or sunflower oil, naturally, it is not going to have any animal fat in it, will it. So there you are, you have 100% animal fat free Fat, which naturally means no cholesterol.

This gimmick was used   by one advertising company in the 90s, and that slogan is now used to advertise cooking fats made up of vegetable oils all over the world. And that is why you are going to buy some expensive cooking oil, which supposedly does not produce any cholesterol in your body.

Olive Oil

For millenniums, people in the Mediterranean region have been distilling olive oil from their juicy, delicious native olives. However, some people dislike the taste, because they are unaccustomed to the flavor. Nevertheless, you can find yourself getting accustomed to its flavor, really well, especially when you begin to use pure olive oil is in your salads and as salad dressing.

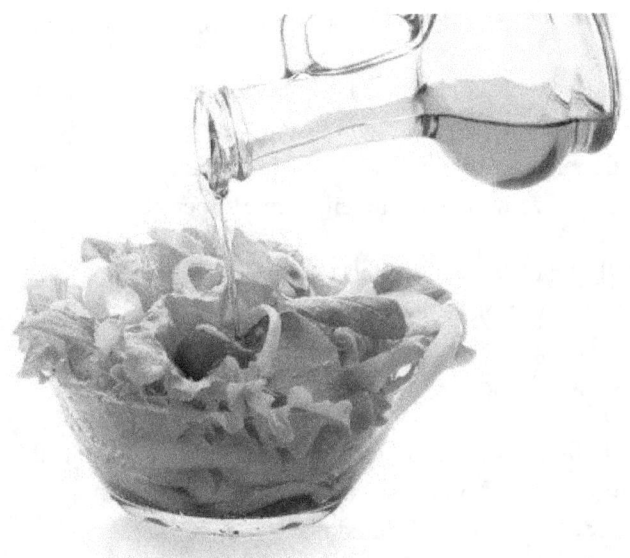

When you get used to the flavor of olive oil, you may want to begin using it for frying.

Olive oil is used extensively as a frying oil, especially when preparing something like a sauce for spaghetti or a dish which originates in the South of France. It is also used for salad dressing and for mayonnaise.

Olive oil is comparatively expensive, and that is why cheaper olive oil, is used in the market, which even though is good for your pocket, is not the real stuff.

When you go shopping for olive oil in the market, you may find plenty of brands available in the market today. But look for extra-virgin olive oil. This is the best quality olive oil for salads. You can use virgin olive oil for frying.

Did you know that 70% of the olive oil being sold as high quality extra-virgin olive oil is fake? That is because it is adulterated with a large number of other oils.

So how do you go checking, which is the best olive oil available in the market today? Unfortunately, Bertolli's and other famous olive oil producers' market standing has taken a beating, because some people decided to test the difference between real olive oil and fake olive oil. So they got a famous importer of olive oil, and some world-famous chefs to taste some olive oil in bowls.

The results were rather shocking. The importer tasted his own imported product, and declared it disgusting! The chefs tasted the olive oil and said they thought it to be really good, high-quality extra-virgin. Well, it just turned out to be an ordinary bottle of virgin olive oil taken from a supermarket shelf.

So if you really want pure olive oil, you will have to go to a supplier who can supply you with the real thing, especially if he has his own family farm with olive groves. There are plenty of these farms in Italy, so you just need to do a little bit of research. And you need to talk directly to them.

Do not buy anything which has a middleman somewhere in the offing. He is going to do a lot of marketing and advertising, and you may find yourself with something of low quality being touted as high quality real stuff.

Coconut Oil

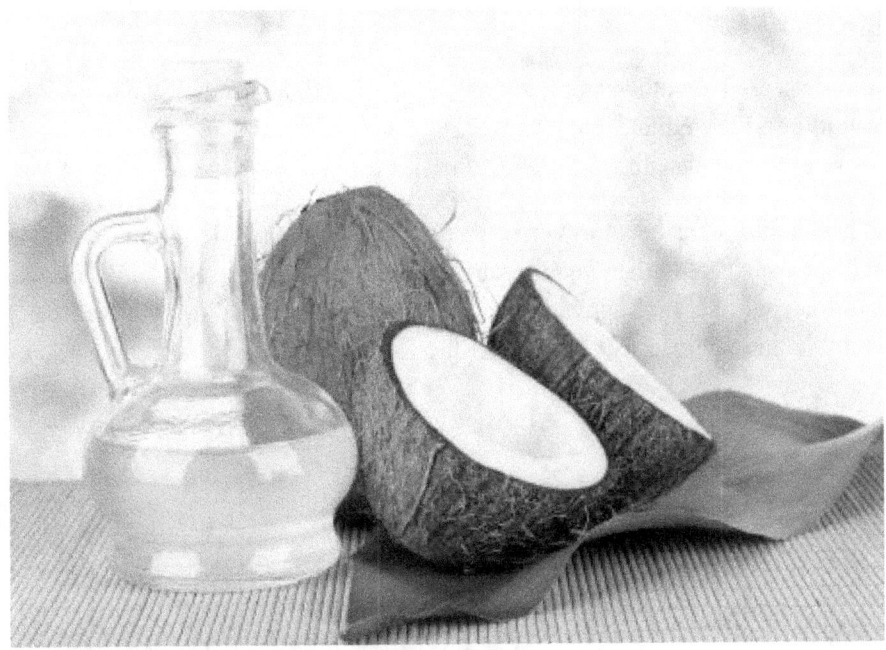

This coconut oil used in beauty treatments, and in spas is quite different from edible coconut oil.

Believe it or not, coconut oil is a major cooking oil, which has been used to centuries, even though many people believe that this product is mainly used as a base for making natural beauty products like moisturizing creams and lotions.

The only problem with coconut oil is that it has a typical nutty flavor. It is finally being discovered as one of the healthiest cooking oils in the world, and people who do not want to eat butter and cream are making their cookies and pastries in coconut oil.

Living most of my life in tropical regions, I was used to coconut oil as a massage oil, since childhood. Apart from that, our traditional and local cook used to fry everything in coconut oil, so we considered it to be a part of our daily cuisine. It was later on that we learned that there were other oils in the world, apart from coconut oil!

Pure coconut oil is stable and healthy and does not go rancid. Philippine cooking as well as people living in the coastal areas of Asia have been using this oil for millenniums.

If you are scared about unsaturated fats and saturated fats, and all the hype surrounding saturated fats and how bad they are for you, it is possible that you do not dare experiment with another new oil.

This is because it has been proven scientifically that not all the saturated fats, which are considered anathema Maranatha and taboo to eat are harmful for you or bad for your health. There are some blood cholesterol raising saturated fats, but they do not necessarily come under the category of bad cholesterol.

Cholesterol

Like all good things, cholesterol is also divided into 2 parts – good cholesterol which is also called HDL – high-density lipoprotein and bad cholesterol, LDL – low-density lipoprotein.

Low density lipoprotein is the cholesterol which is going to go blocking up your arteries and causing potential heart problems. On the other hand, high density lipoprotein is necessary to keep you healthy and your system working properly. That is because it is going to provide plenty of nutritive support to your body, and encourage proper cell functioning and growth.

Coconut oil comes under the good oil category. That is because it has HDL. That means it is actually good for your body. That means any food that you make cooked in coconut oil is going to provide you with plenty of energy. [all right, that was the reason why our teachers and elders could not keep up with us little energetic dynamos. That coconut oil rich diet was to blame…] It is also going to give you a healthy body by raising your metabolic rate.

So if you want to try out coconut oil as a medium of cookery, especially for frying purposes, make sure that you are buying edible coconut oil. This is totally different from coconut hair oil and coconut skin oil.

Refined edible coconut oil can be bought in unrefined and refined form. I preferred the unrefined, because I do not mind the extra strong flavor.

How to know whether you have the real thing or not? Coconut oil is going to be solid at room temperature. It does not turn rancid because it has no polyunsaturated fats in it. If an oil has unsaturated fat content, it is going to turn rancid faster.

Compared to olive oil, coconut oil is cheaper and equally healthy. Also, as it is denser inconsistency, you may find yourself using lesser coconut oil to fry, cook and bake, than when you are using other cooking oils and fats.

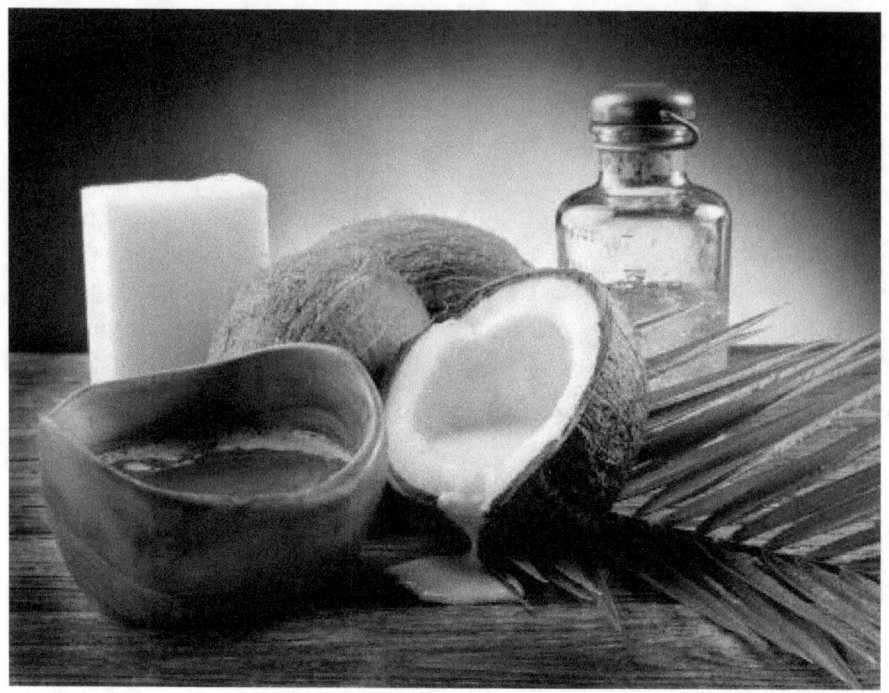

Real unadulterated coconut oil is a soft white vegetable oil, which is semisolid at room temperature, yet melts in response to slight heat. This Pure coconut oil is going to be the color of water.

As it ages, it may start turning yellow, depending upon the amount of impurities left in it. Just place a little bit of coconut oil on your skin, and it should melt instantly. This property is one of the reasons why this oil is used for making preparations, which can be absorbed really quickly after they have been spread in a thin layer all over your skin.

Coconut Butter

Is coconut oil, the same as coconut butter? A number of my friends asked me this question, especially when they were looking for a good base for beauty preparations. The answer is, no, these are two completely different things. Coconut oil is extracted from coconut and so is coconut butter.

How to make Coconut Butter

This butter is a paste, which is made of grinding pieces of coconut flesh with coconut water or with ordinary water. Use pieces of dry coconut, which have been chopped into pieces which can be ground properly in a heavy-duty grinder. Then add some coconut water and grind away to get a paste. It is going to take about 10 – 20 minutes on a heavy-duty grinder, especially when you want a smooth paste.

This is definitely not coconut oil. Coconut oil is obtained by pressing coconuts. It does not have anything to do with the inner nutty portion of a coconut. Coconut butter is a gritty substance and yellowish creamy in color. It is solid at room temperature. It is harder than coconut oil and melts at a much slower rate. That is why it is used for preparing remedies, where slow release of oil is important.

For example, you can use this for making plaisters and suppositories. Suppositories take about ½ to 1 hour to melt, depending on the recipes.

The unique qualities of cocoa butter and coconut oil make them very useful additions to your herbal and beauty product cabinet. You can also use them instead of other fats for making ointments, creams and infusions.

In fact, coconut butter is just about as popular with kids in Asia as a delicious snack spread, as is peanut butter for children in the West. So if you do not have peanut butter around, but have a coconut, try making some cocoa butter and using it as a sandwich spread.

Conclusion

This book gives you information of just a bare minimum of the popular fats and all used for cooking and for other purposes, all over the world. There are of course other cooking fatty mediums like sesame oil, mustard oil and so on, depending on the easily availability of these products in your area or locality.

Nevertheless, knowing a little bit of these oils and fats and their importance in keeping your system healthy and functioning properly, make sure that at least some fatty foods are a part of your daily diet.

Why did not I write about polyunsaturated fats and saturated fats, and all those other scary scientific syllables, you may ask? That is because I am writing a book giving you important and useful information. I am not writing about something which is full of controversies, scientific research statistics, heated discussions, and other tiresome and often misleading information.

There is a person coming out with a new theory every day. One fine day, you may find somebody with a number of Degrees to his name telling you that real honest to goodness, homemade butter is excellent for your health. And you are going to see an important film star endorsing the goodness of butter. Then wait for the sales of homemade butter, going up.

On the other hand, someone is going to say that margarine is terrible for health, or the butter oil exported from European countries to other parts of the world is contaminated with nuclear waste[3] and you are going to see everybody shunning margarine or butter – oil like the plague.

---

[3] Real Fact – Millions of tons of very high quality butter oil exported to India from Europe in the early 80s, was immediately boycotted because this rumor went up that they had sent us radioactive nuclear waste contaminated food, which had been condemned by their own government. Otherwise, why would they want to sell it to us at such affordable prices, when they had never done it before? There was something rotten in the state of Denmark, no pun intended.

We were taking no chances. So our then government canceled all those contracts, especially the import of very high-quality butter oil from Sweden and Denmark. But one

Use your own judgment. Eat healthy, eat in limited quantities, and eat sensibly.
Live Long and Prosper!

still remembers with fond nostalgia, the high-quality of that butter oil and its delicious
taste.

Author Bio-

Dueep Jyot Singh is a Management and IT Professional who managed to gather Postgraduate qualifications in Management and English and Degrees in Science, French and Education while pursuing different enjoyable career options like being an hospital administrator, IT,SEO and HRD Database Manager/ trainer, movie , radio and TV scriptwriter, theatre artiste and public speaker, lecturer in French, Marketing and Advertising, ex-Editor of Hearts On Fire (now known as Solstice) Books Missouri USA, advice columnist and cartoonist, publisher and Aviation School trainer, ex- moderator on Medico.in, banker, student councilor ,travelogue writer … among other things!

One fine morning, she decided that she had enough of killing herself by Degrees and went back to her first love -- writing. It's more enjoyable! She already has 48 published academic and 14 fiction- in- different- genre books under her belt.

When she is not designing websites or making Graphic design illustrations for clients , she is browsing through old bookshops hunting for treasures, of which she has an enviable collection – including R.L. Stevenson, O.Henry, Dornford Yates, Maurice Walsh, De Maupassant, Victor Hugo, Sapper, C.N. Williamson, "Bartimeus" and the crown of her collection- Dickens "The Old Curiosity Shop," and so on… Just call her "Renaissance Woman") - collecting herbal remedies, acting like Universal Helping Hand/Agony Aunt, or escaping to her dear mountains for a bit of exploring, collecting herbs and plants and trekking.

1. Amazon.com
2. Barnes and Noble
3. Itunes
4. Kobo
5. Smashwords
6. Google Play Books

Check out some of the other JD-Biz Publishing books

Gardening Series on Amazon

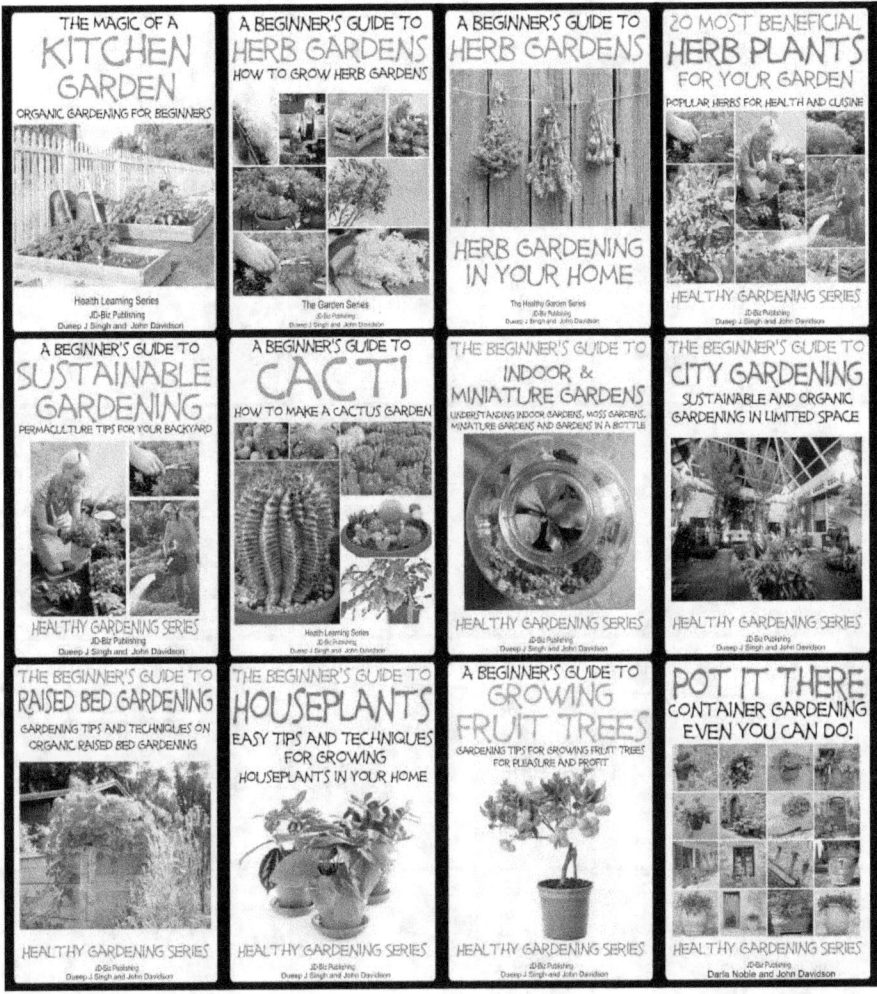

Health Learning Series

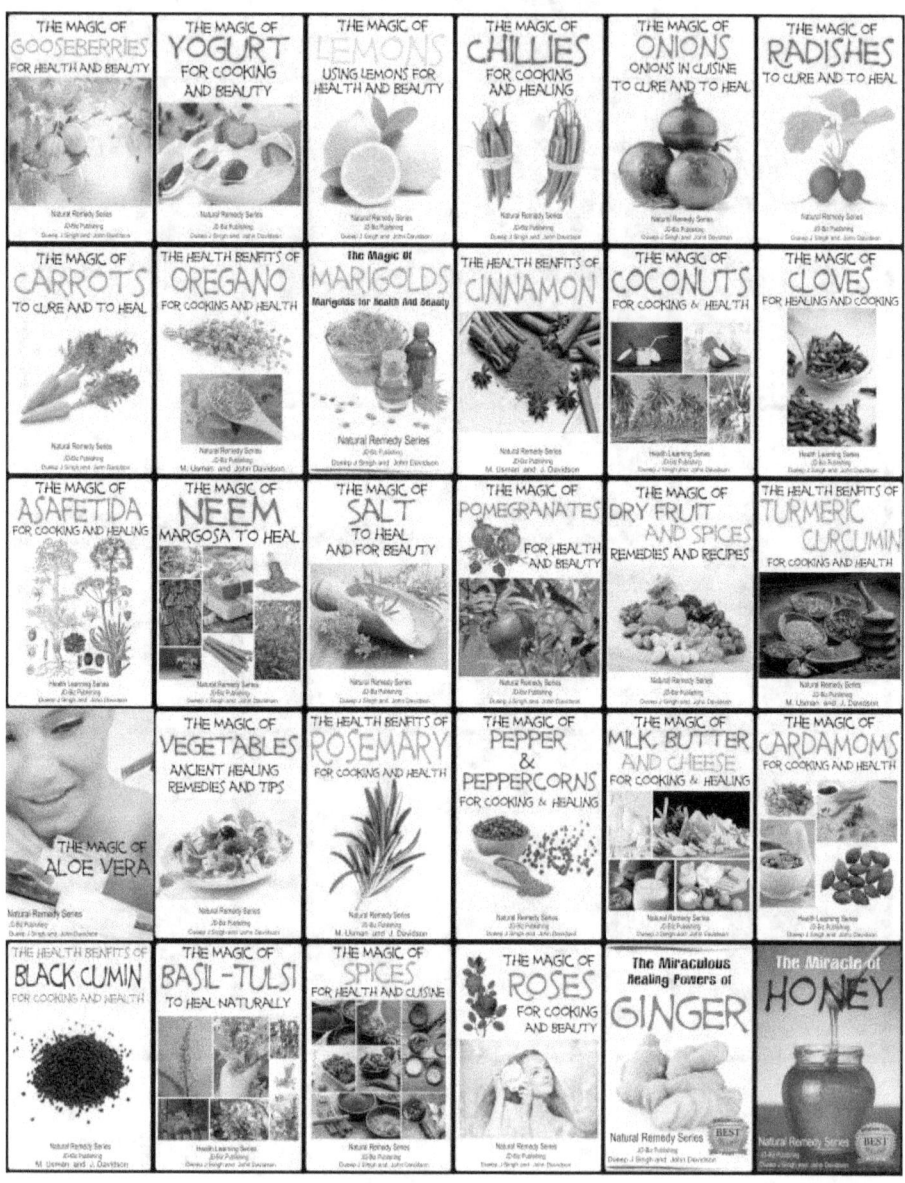

Country Life Books

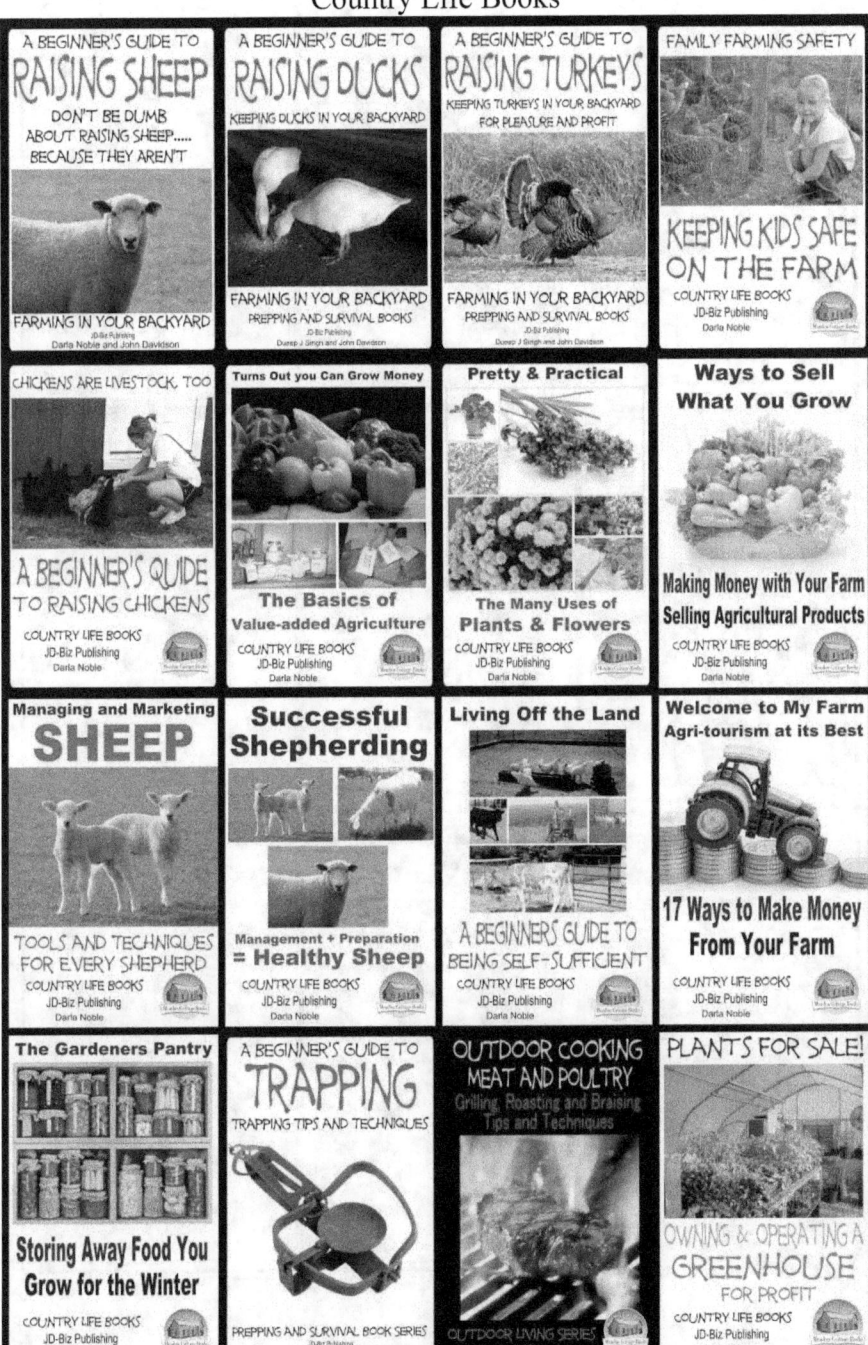

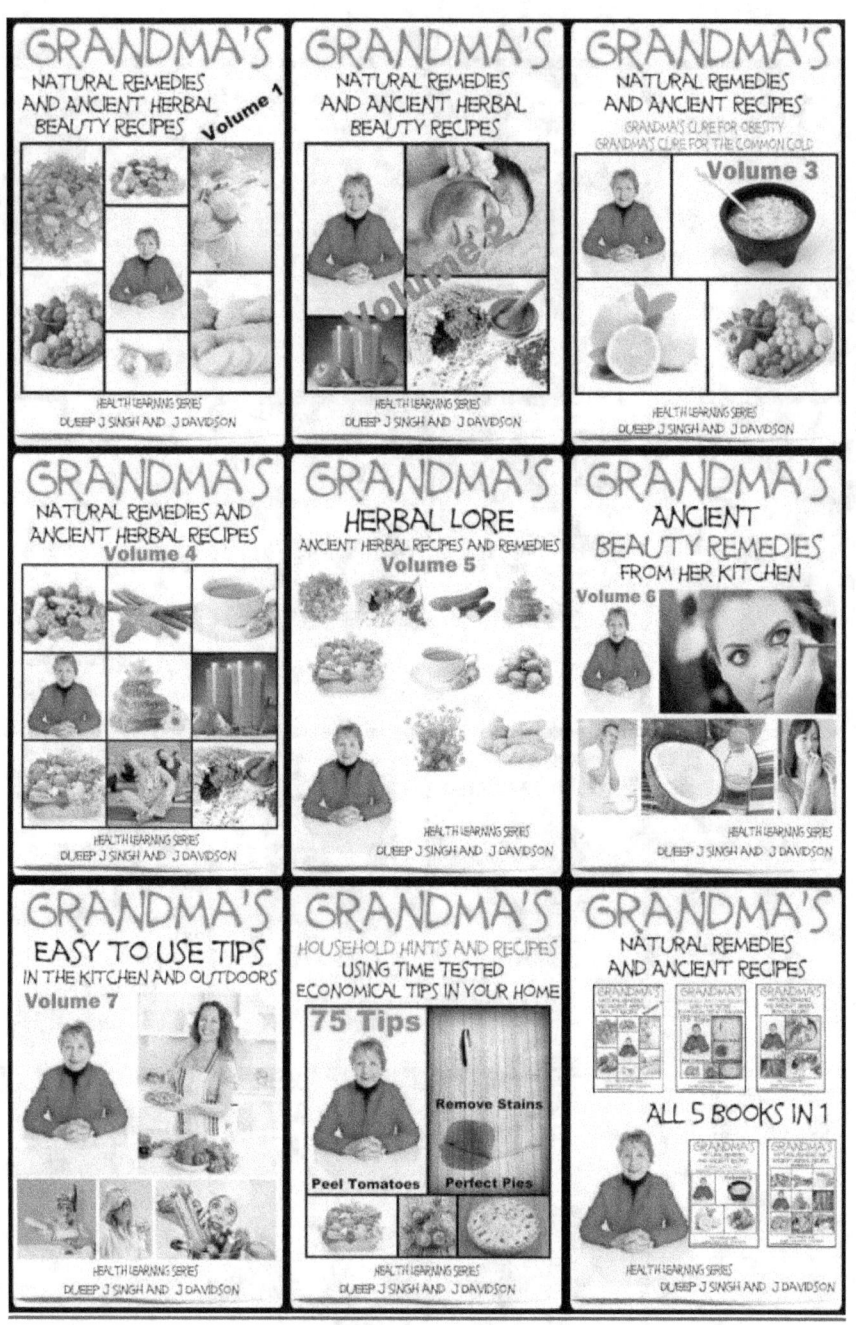

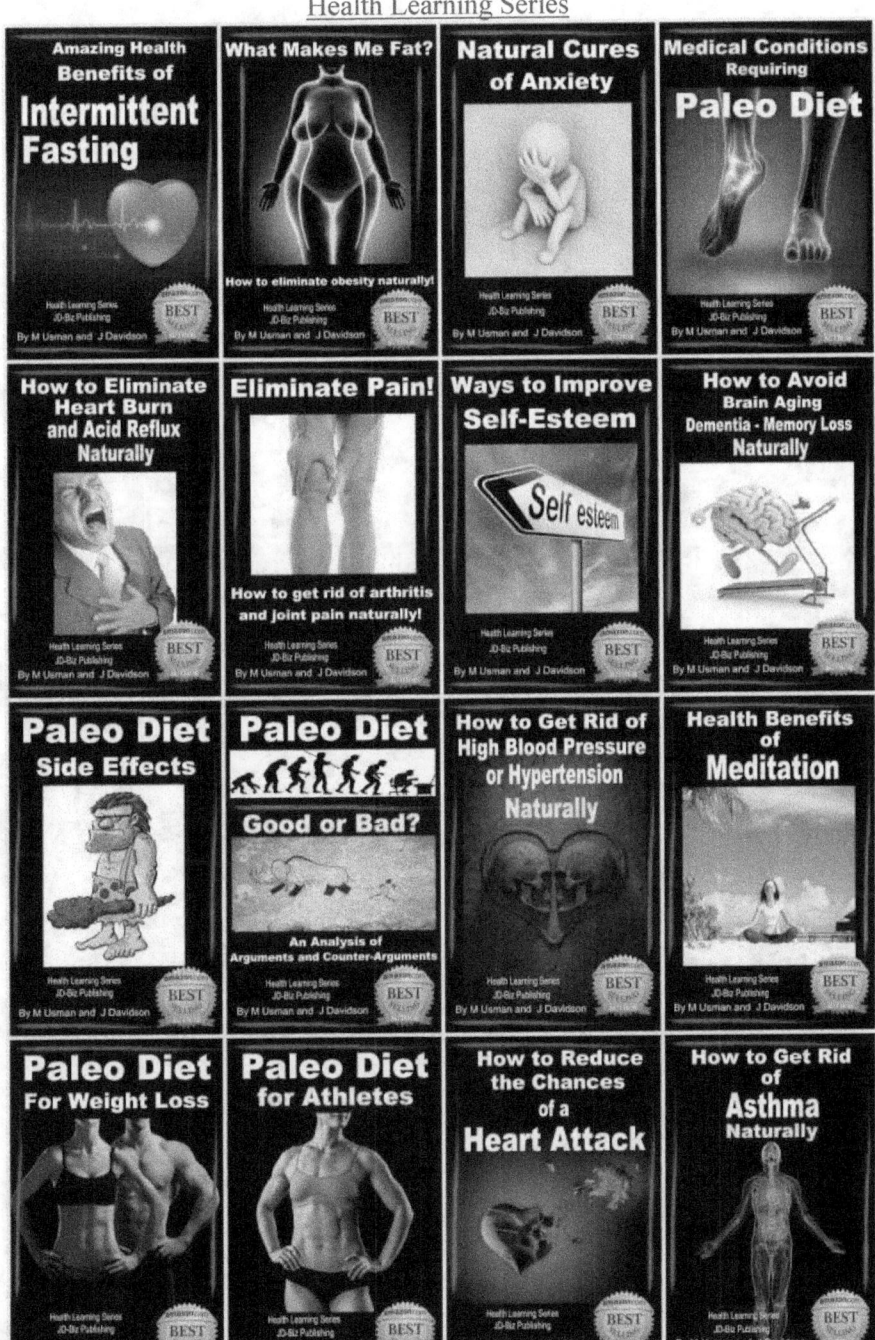

Amazing Animal Book Series

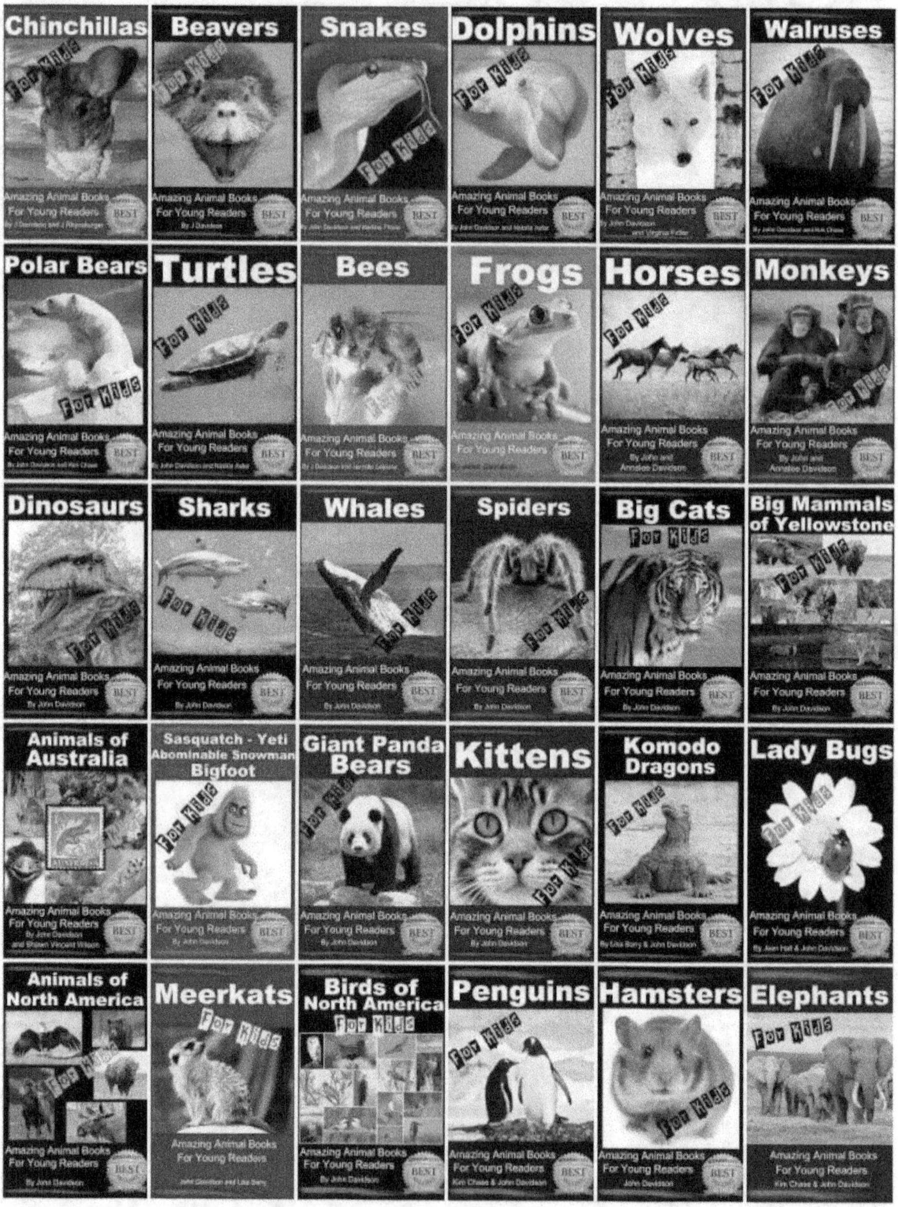

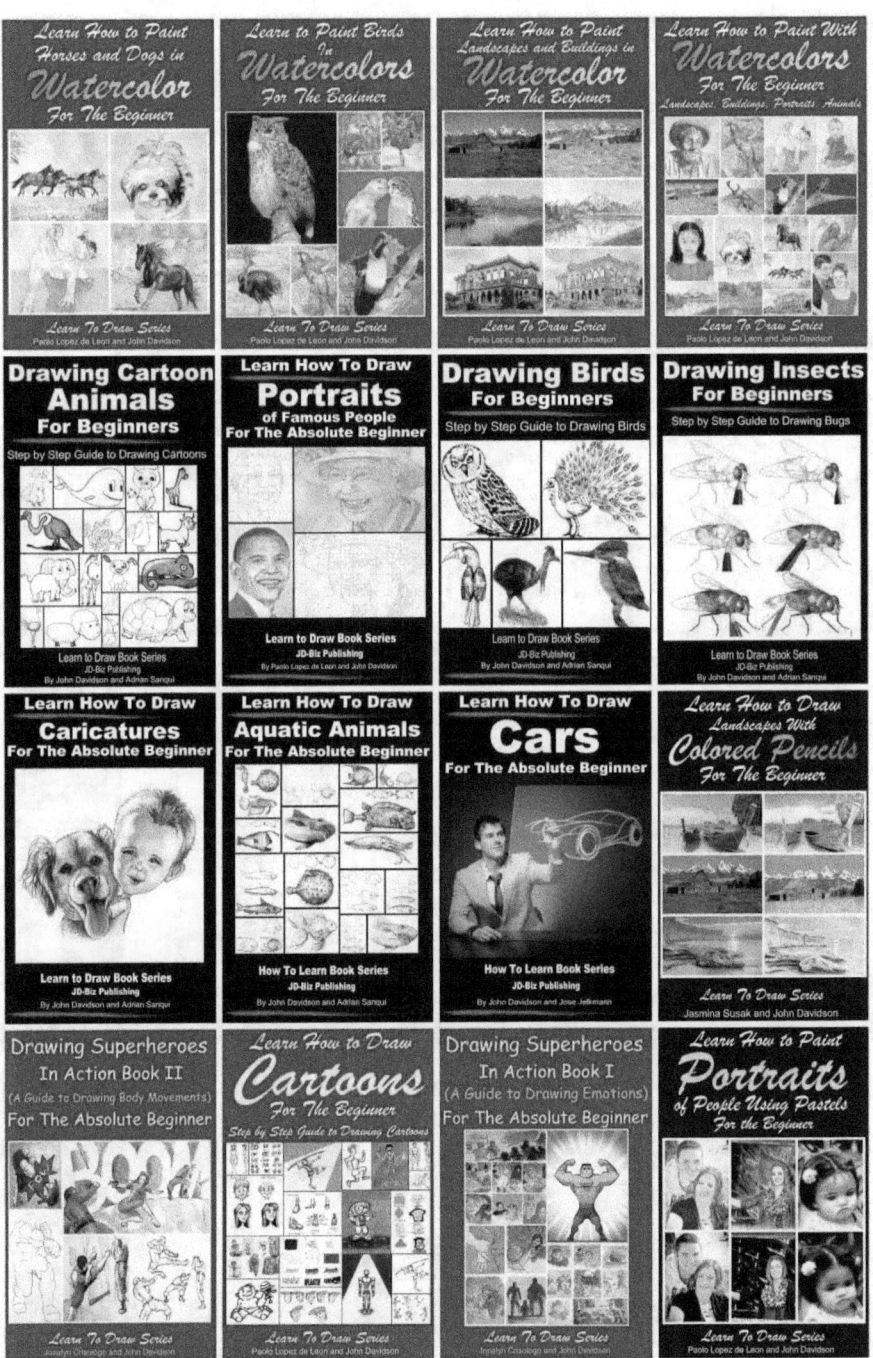

How to Build and Plan Books

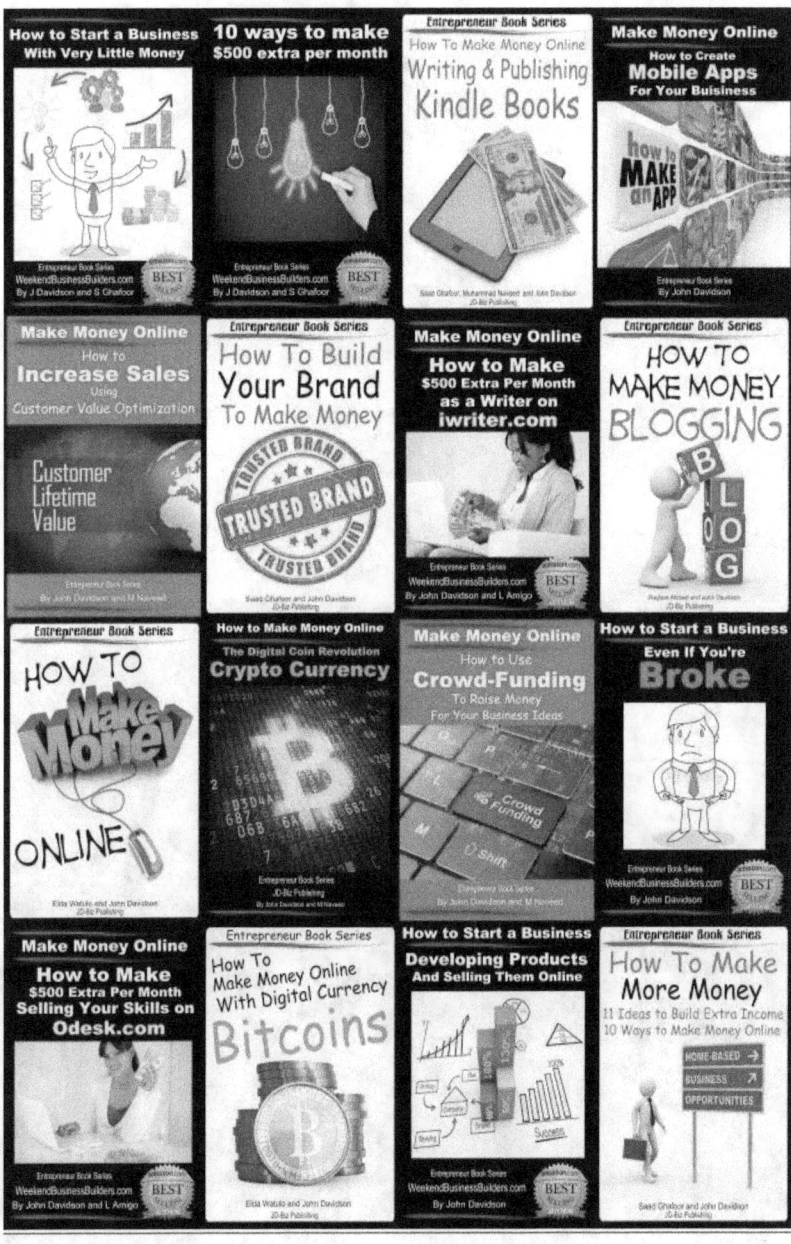

Publisher

JD-BIZ
PUBLISHING

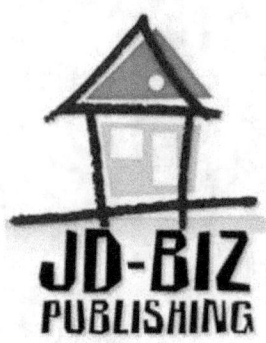

JD-Biz Corp

P O Box 374

Mendon, Utah 84325

http://www.jd-biz.com/

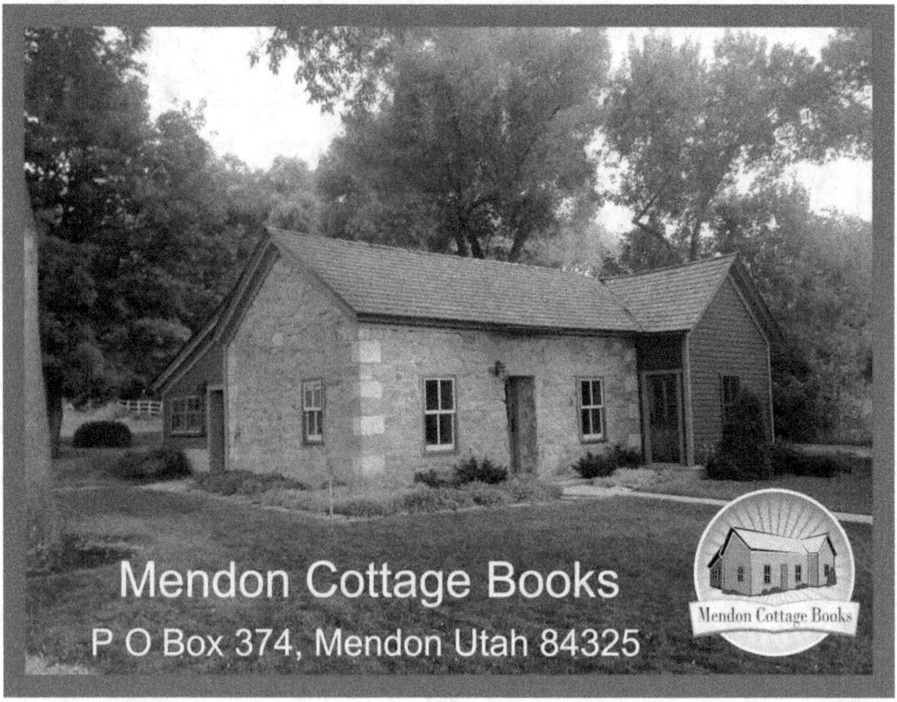

Mendon Cottage Books
P O Box 374, Mendon Utah 84325
Mendon Cottage Books